No one is Perfect
and Y♥U
are a Great Kid

Kim Hix

This book is dedicated to all of the children in the world who desperately want to fit in but feel different, isolated or rejected. To all the wonderful, loving, special children who suffer from behavioral or mood disorders, depression or mental illness, for having to endure and live among those who don't understand. To my dear husband for indulging my wild ideas and supporting my projects, for making me laugh when I want to cry. To my loving, dear Zack, you endure so much, yet love so deep, for trying so hard and facing each day hoping for a miracle. You will be great, you will make it, you will succeed. To my sweet Kelsie, for living among the chaos and bringing smiles and laughter to us all. To my parents, for simply being who they are, for being wonderful, supportive and dependable, my love for you is immeasurable. To Dr. Richards for giving us hope when we thought there was none. Finally, to Lee Dillingham, for bringing my story to life, you are the most talented person I have ever met. Thank you all.

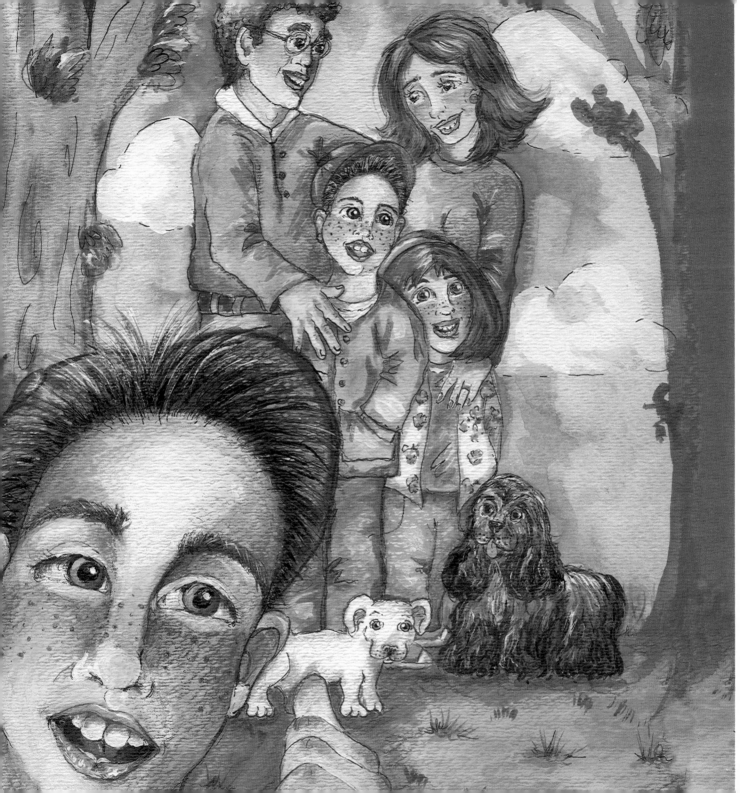

Hi, my name is Zack. I am 10 years old. I love to have fun, play with friends, swim, play games and spend time with my family. I have two dogs and a sister; my life is pretty normal, except that I feel different from my friends. Feeling different is hard for a kid. A kid can feel different in a lot of ways. For example, you may feel different in how you look, talk or act. You may even feel like your family is not like most others. Do you ever feel different from your friends or classmates? I would like to tell you how I feel different.

No one is perfect......

You are a great kid

Most days are good and fun for me, but some days can be very hard and frustrating. My emotions can be like a roller coaster ride. I can get very upset and mad at little things. Well, it may seem little to some people but they seem really big to me and I don't understand why. Does that ever happen to you? Then I get mad at myself and mom says to me, "It's ok Zack, "No one is perfect and you are a great kid."

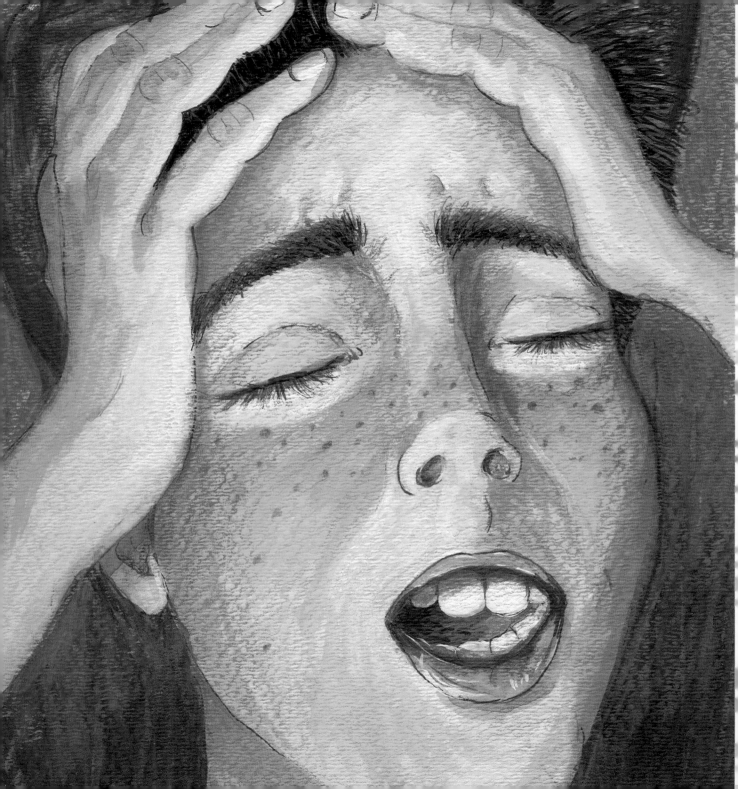

When I get angry or upset it feels like my head is on fire and I can't control it or make myself calm down. A lot of times, things make me mad that would not make my friends or other people upset. For example, just the other day I was playing football and we were choosing teams. The other boys wanted me on the team with the little kids!!! I did not think that was fair!!! So I got upset and then my friends didn't want me to play anymore. That hurt my feelings. I really wanted to play and have fun.

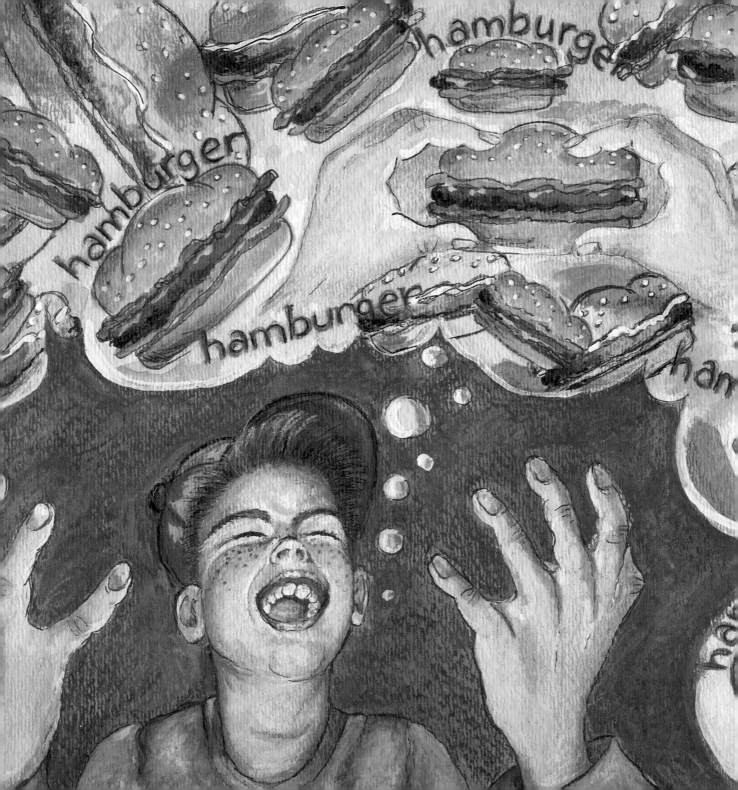

♡ne day last week, I was having a great time with my family. I got hungry and wanted a hamburger from my favorite restaurant, but my mom said "no" because I already had one that week. I REALLY wanted a hamburger! That's all I could think about. The thought of that hamburger would not go away. Mom kept saying "not today", so I started yelling and kicking things. I got angrier and angrier. I was very disrespectful to my parents and would not listen to them. Doesn't that sound like a silly reason to get so mad? My fit lasted a long time, maybe an hour. I tried to calm down but I just couldn't. Mom calls these my "episodes". She says something takes over me. Boy, did I get in trouble.

I hate to get into trouble. Sometimes when I do things I shouldn't, mom takes my favorite toy, or won't let me play with my friends. I keep hoping I will learn to make better choices and to control my angry feelings so that I won't get into trouble so much. I try very hard to control my angry moods. Guess what? I'm getting better at managing my feelings. When mom and I talk about it she reminds me that "No one is perfect and you are a great kid." Even when I do things that I should not do.

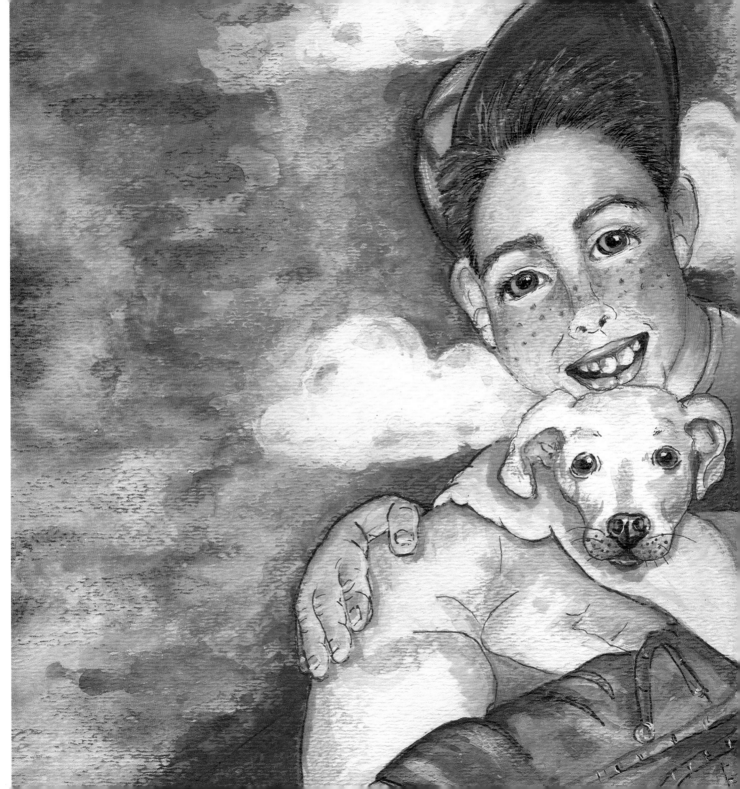

When I get my mind set on something, it's all I can think about. Mom tries to help me think of other things but I just can't. It's like my brain gets stuck on one thing and it lasts forever. It is kind of like a song you hear and you sing it all day long. It's terrible to feel this way. Especially when I want something really bad and I can't stop thinking about it, or try to draw something or complete something perfectly. I just can't stop, no matter how hard I try. I wonder, am I the only kid that has this problem?

I always feel real sorry for how I have acted towards my friends and family when I say mean things to them. I know I should not have done them. Most people don't understand that I try to be good, that I really am a good boy. They just seem to remember when I do things that I shouldn't. Mom talks to me about it and says remember "No one is perfect and you are a great kid." She understands.

My mom says sometimes it seems like two boys are living in my body because when I feel good I am the sweetest boy in the world. Then the days when I am mad and in a "mood" or have so much energy that I can't stop moving....watch out. It can be a very long day for everybody. It feels like the day will never end. I just want the day to be over so I can wake up and start a new day, hopefully a better day.

Just when I thought things could not get any worse, my face started making strange movements, all on its own. My tongue started sticking out, my nose would crinkle and my eyes would blink. It was very annoying, and boy did that give the other kids something else to pick on me about. Mom said these are tics, and thank goodness they have become less noticeable over time.

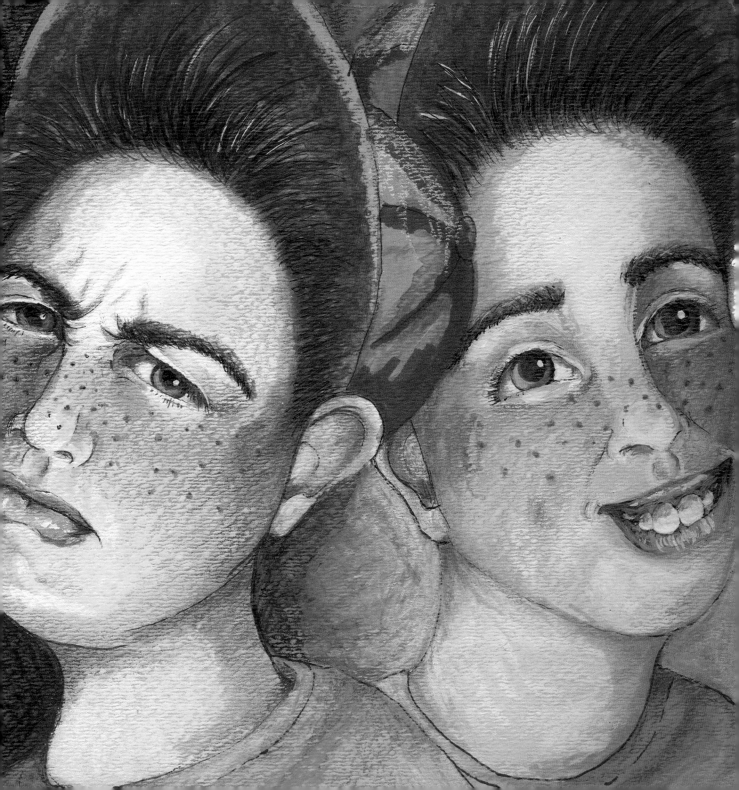

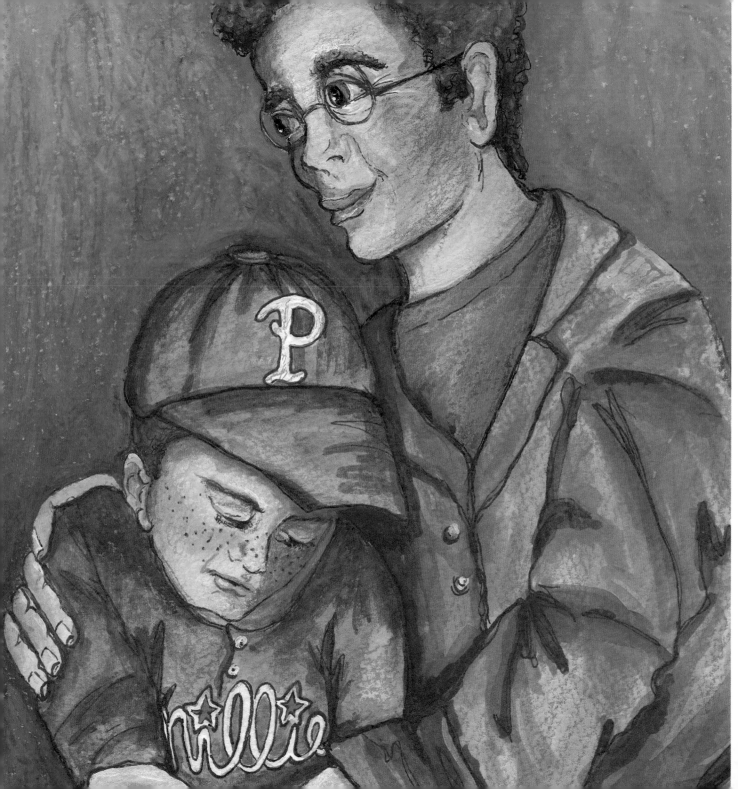

I get sad sometimes too. I cry a lot, my feelings get hurt easily and I feel rotten. I feel like I don't deserve to be part of my family. I feel different and wonder why. I think I am the only kid who has these problems. Why do I get so mad? Why do I get so sad? Do other kids feel bad like I do? Then mom says "No one is perfect and you are a great kid."

Mom tells me I have to learn to make better choices and I have to work harder than other kids at most things, like being patient and not getting upset. She also tells me that the things that upset and frustrate me now, like my need to be perfect, and to always win or be the best can make me a great and successful adult. I sure hope she is right.

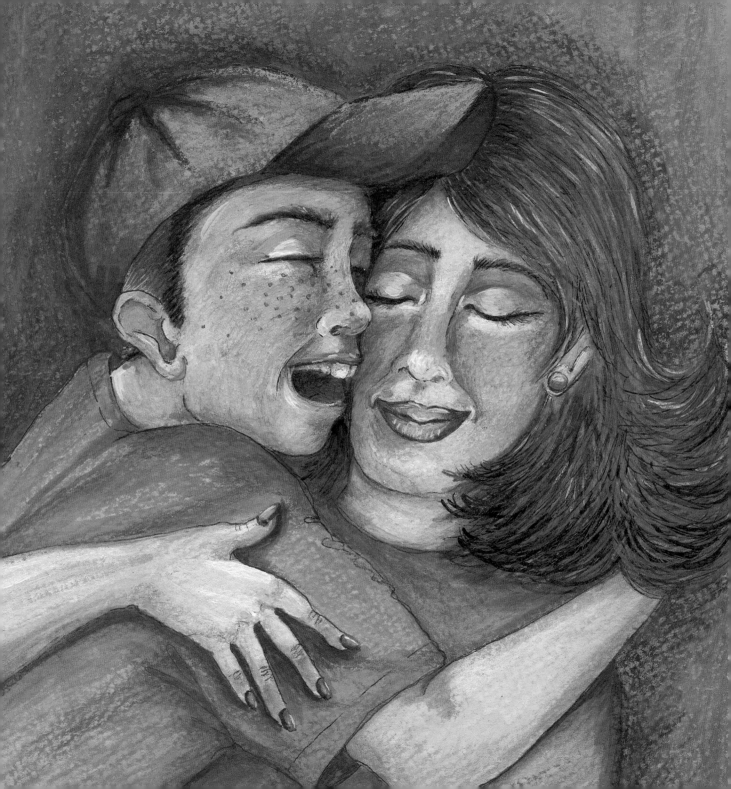

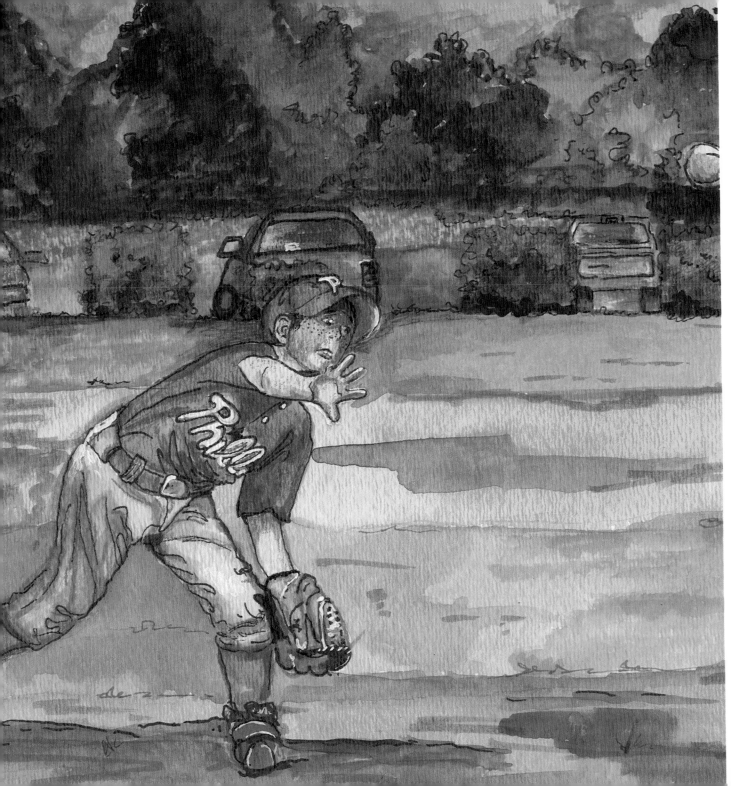

I am a really good baseball player and good at most sports. I love to throw football and baseball with my dad. That's what I want to be when I grow up, a professional baseball player. My parents tell me I am a natural athlete and that is my gift. I can also draw some cool pictures.

You should know great kids come in all shapes, sizes, colors and nationalities. We all just want to fit in, have friends and enjoy life. If Y♡U want to be something or do something then you just have to keep trying and never give up. Mom says that Impossible is just a word that doesn't mean anything unless you want it to. Everyone has a gift; you just have to find it. Have you found your gift yet? What do you enjoy doing?

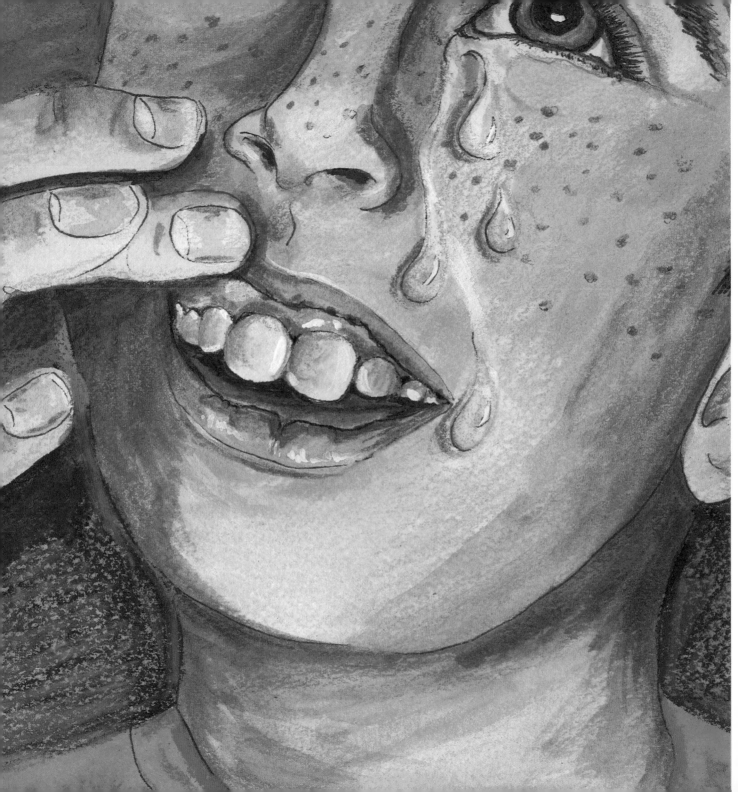

Some days when I'm in a bad mood nothing seems right. Everything aggravates me and makes me mad. My socks feel funny, my clothes don't feel good or my food tastes bad. I think my teeth are too big and my stomach is fat. I yell at my sister and the dog. It's just a bad day. I think I am a bad boy until mom says, remember "no one is perfect and you are a great kid."

I can make things real hard for my family, but they love me anyway. I don't mean to make things hard for them, but sometimes that other boy in my body takes over and I can't make him go away. I try to, but some days the bad mood stays. I wonder why the other kids seem so perfect, why can't I be? It seems like they do everything right. They never get in time out, and they never get into trouble. Like my sister, she seems perfect in every way. Then mom will remind me that "No one is perfect and you are a great kid"

Sometimes being a kid is hard, especially when you feel different, whether you look different, act different or talk different. Mom says that the world is made up of all kinds of different people because that is what makes the world an interesting place. Wouldn't it be boring if we were all the same? But just because you may be different or feel different doesn't mean you can't have fun or don't enjoy playing with friends or learning new things. You are great just how YOU are. So just remember...

"No one is perfect and you are a great kid."

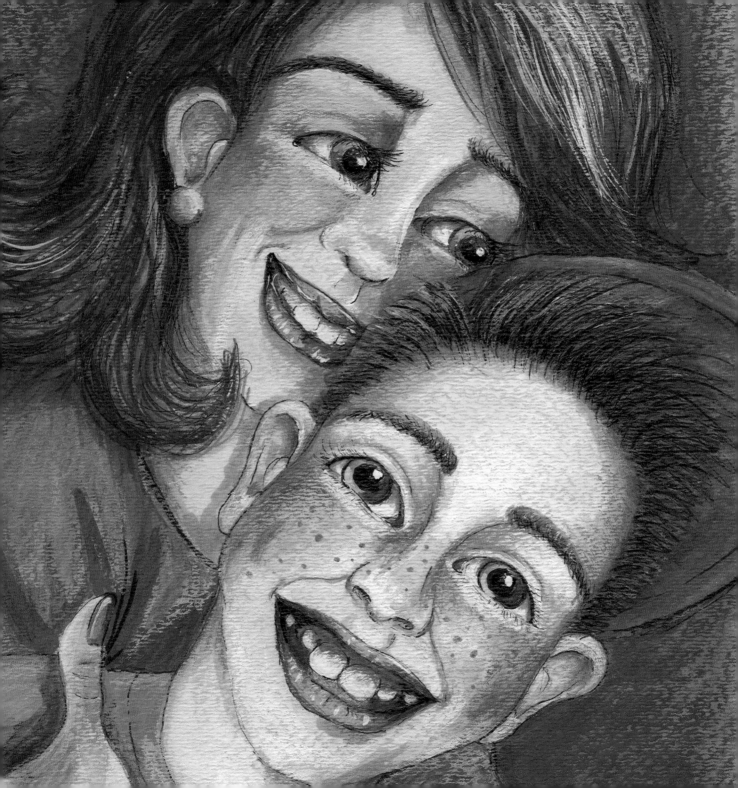

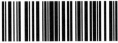

Made in the USA
Charleston, SC
04 November 2010